It Just Got Real

The Secret Scoop of Early Motherhood

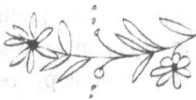

SARAH WORKMAN CHECCONE

Excerpt from Bump to Grind: The Secret Scoop on Labor, Delivery, and Early Motherhood

Praeclarus Press, LLC

www.PraeclarusPress.com

Praeclarus Press, LLC

2504 Sweetgum Lane

Amarillo, Texas 79124 USA

806-367-9950

www.PraeclarusPress.com

DISCLAIMER

The information contained in this publication is advisory only
and is not intended to replace sound clinical judgment or indi-
vidualized patient care. The author disclaims all warranties,
whether expressed or implied, including any warranty as the
quality, accuracy, safety, or suitability of this information for
any particular purpose.

ISBN: 978-1-946665-02-7

Cover Design: Ken Tackett

Developmental Editing: Kathleen Kendall-Tackett

Copyediting: Chris Tackett

Layout & Design: Nelly Murariu

Contents

Preface

This book was written for you, First Time Mothers. To reduce your stress as you adjust to motherhood, ease your birth/postpartum transition, and put some peer support in the palm of your hand. Literally. After all, moms weren't meant to do this alone.

If you are pregnant or have a baby under 12 months, you are in the "Perinatal Period," and likely in the midst of the most significant life transition you'll ever experience. A lot goes down in those 21 months from conception to baby's first birthday, including many things we never, ever expected.

When we, as moms-to-be, prepare to bring baby home, we have certain dreams and expectations. We buy things, read books, take classes, and politely nod (usually) as advice and anecdotes are heaped upon us. We focus on making it through pregnancy and giving birth, and imagine our maternal instincts will take over when our little cutie is in our arms. Preparing for baby is so important, both logistically and psychologically, but there's another new person coming home after delivery, too. A new mother.

As new (postpartum) mothers, our wellness is crucial to the whole new-baby operation getting off the ground, and if we have to juggle taking care of a newborn *while* trying to figure out the unexpected physical and mental complexities of birth and post-partum, it's just too much. This extra processing requires additional emotional energy and adds post-partum stress to an already exhausted new mom's plate—right when she needs to focus on her own and her baby's wellness. The more I speak with new mothers, the more I am certain a lack of open, honest communication about birth and the post-partum process is seriously counterproductive–even dangerous–to maternal and infant health.

If women in the perinatal period have real infor-mation about birth and postpartum-related issues that could and commonly do arise (though they are rarely discussed), they can reduce their post-partum stress and lessen their risk for postpartum distress (depression, anxiety, etc.). No one can be prepared for every scenario, but what if a new mom could "expect the unexpected" to some degree? For example, what if a new mom could know...

♥ Many new mothers have stressful hospital stays.

♥ A lot of women don't feel the immediate bond with their babies that they expected.

♥ A majority of new moms feel frustrated and angry that their own lives have changed much more than their partners.'

♥ It's common for a new mom to feel a loss of her own identity and really miss her old self and her old freedom in the first year of motherhood

If she knew these truths and more, maybe she wouldn't feel as afraid, alone, or experience a sense of failure when motherhood isn't quite (or at all) what she expected. Perhaps, she'd feel more comfortable reaching out to someone for support. Real stories help to normalize the abnormal, and when the going gets tough, that window to reality can be a light in a new mother's darkness.

The miracle of sharing real stories and experiences with other new moms is the normalizing of the abnormal (to a reasonable degree—not explaining away the harmful or dysfunctional). When postpartum women get together with other new moms, listen, and share their realities, they understand they are not alone in their challenges. Suddenly, a mom in distress doesn't feel like such a "failure" or a "bad mother" anymore. She's just a real mother, with ups and downs like anyone else, doing the best she can.

No matter what you experience as a new mother, please know *you are not alone*. Maybe knowing that is enough for you to deal with the rough stuff and move on, but when the chips are down, face-to-face connection with other women who can relate can be incredibly valuable.

In our Postpartum Support Group, we frequently discuss what we wish we'd known before we gave birth. Then, one day, a group member said to me, "You should write a book about all this stuff—it could really help some new moms." I had to laugh, because that's exactly what I was doing. There's a clear connection between shock and distress. The information in this book aims to lessen some of the shocks of the peak of the perinatal period in order to reduce your stress and distress. And to give you a good laugh, too. Enjoy, and all the best to you, your partner, and your baby!

POSTPARTUM ADJUSTMENT

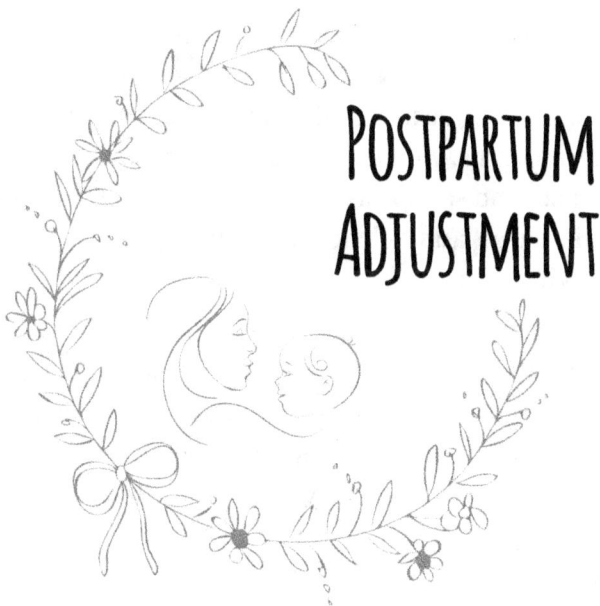

It Just Got Real

I knew the postpartum period would not be glamorous, but I had no effing idea. I knew I'd be crazy, but again, no effing idea. I don't think there's any way to really prepare for it other than to know it's a hell of a ride, and there are a few things that might help, or mean you need some help.

ANGIE G.

So now you're home, and everything feels unstable and shifty at the moment. That's because it is. If you try to understand it, question it, or worry about it too much, it may only scare you. You are now in the postpartum phase, outside of hospital recovery, removed from the birth experience, but still in a "Fourth Trimester" with your baby. For the next few months, your baby still needs your body, touch, smell, and sounds as something of a shield against the harsh and relentless stimuli of his/her new environment.

Whether you want to talk about your feelings, write about them (chat boards and Facebook pages are great venting spots), or wave your anxieties away, many new moms look back at early post-partum and agree that you can't really understand the massive feelings and changes in the days (and weeks and months) after birth. Similar to adolescence, it just starts, and you do your best to hang on without losing your grip. But know this—you are not flying solo, Mama. There are lots of us clinging to the rear bumper of motherhood right along with you, and we're all in this together.

Redefining Power and Control

When mom brings baby home, she may feel a seismic shift in the world she once (mostly) controlled, felt free in and understood. After birth, everything changes so quickly, she can feel completely overwhelmed and power-less. To stabilize and move forward, she may need to temporarily redefine "power" and "control," so she doesn't feel emotionally and mentally flattened.

When a baby comes home, everything changes, and for awhile things may feel somewhat (or totally) out of control. But please know this: *you still have power and control, just in a different form.* Each of us has the power to be kind to ourselves, to nourish ourselves with good thoughts, such as, "I am a good person. I don't have to be 'perfect' to be good," and "This is really hard, and it will get easier. I am working really, really hard and doing a good job." And you are.

As new mothers, even though everything can feel out of control at times, we do have power and control in our worlds:the power to control ourselves. If we don't feel able to control ourselves, we still have the power to reach out for help to find a new sense of control and empowerment. As we say to our kids when they're in school, "You can only control yourself. We can do our best not to let others' behavior and moods control you."

Even as a perfect storm of exhaustion, isolation, and upheaval rages around us, and threatens to invade our hearts and minds, we still have power and control– the power to listen to and trust our instincts, draw boundaries and counter self-destructive inner monologues with positive thoughts and actions, and reach out for the support we need. There are so many women who understand and are there for new moms as they transition, whatever the situation. There's safety in numbers, Mama. You do not need to go through this transition alone.

Getting Back to "Normal"

My postpartum period with my daughter is a total blur. I hardly remember anything about her first year. I guess that's nature's way of ensuring the propagation of the species. If we remembered how much a lot of this sucks, we wouldn't keep going back for more!

SELMA G.

Once you and baby are home, you may be anxious to get back to normal. Normal you, normal partner. Sure, you know the sleeping thing is going to be tough for a while, but everything else? It really shouldn't be *that* shaken up. After all, you only brought home a baby. People do that every day in every country in the world, so what's the big deal, right? *Right?* I'm just going to get back to *normal. Normal, dammit!!! NORMAL!!!!! AHHHHHH!!!!!!!*

It was healthy to get that out. Yes, the desire to get back to "normal," whether it's following the birth of your first, second, or tenth child, is very, well, *normal.* We often don't realize how drastically something is about to change, or has changed, until well after the fact. Then, there's no road back, only forward. Time to find a New Normal.

Taking Care of You

So, you and I have now weathered some pretty huge moments together, so are you willing to do something, even if it's just to humor me? Will you please consider letting go of any latent beliefs that it's somehow indulgent or self-centered to prioritize taking care of yourself? Feel free to write a note to this effect, and tape it to your baby's changing table, where you can read it routinely. I found out the hard way that putting myself dead last is a recipe for disaster, and am now a true believer in the power of inexpensive, yet effective, Take-Care-of-Mom techniques, such as vertical hydrotherapy and boxed multi-meal solutions. (Also known as "showers" and "cereal," respectively).

Hopefully, others are available to take care of you at this time, too. Some new moms employ post-partum doulas, and appreciate their wrap-around style of support (visit www.dona.org to find a certified doula near you). If a doula isn't an option, and you don't have others to help you during your postpartum recovery (many women don't–grandmothers who can't be present, husbands who work all the time, stress in the family and more), *you have got to be in charge of taking care of* **you** *first. You, as the mother, are the bedrock of the family, and* **when you take care of yourself, you are taking care of your baby and family, too.** In early motherhood, there are some corners you can cut, and some you can't, but *YOU* are never a corner to be cut, Mama. You are the center of the whole operation.

I don't mean to sound bossy, I only aim to plant a seed of permission so when you are home with your baby and 10 free minutes appear, and you can choose to either fold the laundry, or watch something funny on TV and eat with two hands, I hope you'll allow yourself to take a break *without feeling guilty*. Mothers at home with little ones need lots of breaks, even teeny breaks–no babysitters required. For example, going into a different room for a little while and reading, or sitting on the front step breathing deeply for 5 minutes. If you recall, folks in the workplace take lots of breaks–big and small–and have people to talk to. Just because you're home does *not* mean you have any free time.

A mom has to choose to take those momentary breaks for herself, for her own sanity.

Expectations and "Enjoying the Baby"

In my humble opinion, the first 3 months have some sweet moments, but overall they are the total pits. Just remember, they're not predictive of the future. They're the uphill part of the postpartum marathon. They aren't the "Motherhood Experience." There are lots of times that it's more than okay to just put your head down and get through it.

RAINA C.

Oh Lord, expectations. We all have them, and they can really screw with our heads. The expectations we have of ourselves as mothers, our partners as fathers, our babies, and all our dearest maternal fantasies can be a lot to face, and even more to let go of. Often our expectations of motherhood revolve around how well (we believe) we will understand our babies. We also may have expectations of ourselves to be "perfect" mothers: endlessly calm, energetic, and patient. We may have had this type of mother-figure in our lives, or we may have only imagined such a person based on women we knew or works of fiction, but the origin of our expectations matter less than simply understanding these are dreams and images only. They may inspire us or make us feel like failures, but these expectations are not a reasonable measuring stick of whether we are "good mothers."

Another common expectation of motherhood is that we, as mothers, will "enjoy the baby." Right. After we've been torn from stem to stern, are adjusting to status as a food source and the accompanying razor-blade gums, not to mention coping with levels of sleep deprivation that would make grown men cry. You may, in fact, have film footage to illustrate this point.

What does "enjoy the baby" even mean? Enjoy the overall experience? Enjoy every minute? That's, as my 5-year-old says, "Totally nutso-banana cakes." People say "Enjoy the baby" because they *wish* they had enjoyed their babies, not because it's actually *possible to* enjoy newbornhood, or even early motherhood. Enjoying sweet moments, and taking some video may be as good as it gets. Much of raising little children is hard and repetitive work. That's why the good Lord made them so cute. One mother of two put it this way:

> *Enjoy the baby. Duh, right? Except nothing about parenting, not from the first minute, will be exactly what you want or expect. And at some point, especially if you are crazy with postpartum hormones (and I guarantee you will be looney, it goes with the territory), you will fixate on whatever*

those little imperfect things are, and they will take over your life.

If you remind yourself that it's about the baby, and enjoying those precious, brief moments of newbornhood, some of that noise will fade into the background. I know it's not the same for everyone. So much of my daughter's early newbornhood was exactly the opposite of what I imagined, and the only thing that got me through was reminding myself to enjoy the baby. I would repeat it to myself over and over, like a mantra.

ANGIE G.

Maternity Leave

The U.S. is the only industrialized country without paid maternity leave. The reality of maternity leave tends to be a cruel joke. A mom of two captured the essence:

Maternity leave will not be a break. You will not get the chance to catch up on projects at home. You will not have "free time." I thought I'd have loads of free time. I laugh hysterically at my naive self. Maybe someone else could have swung it. I considered myself a gold-star mama when I got a shower that didn't somehow involve me running across the bedroom, dripping wet, to soothe the baby.

ANGIE G.

Several other moms agreed:

Just accept that you will be constantly exhausted at least in the first 6 weeks, if not the first 6 months, when the sleep starts to stretch out at night. Do NOT try to "catch up" on scrapbooking, basement cleaning, that book you were writing, or any other big projects during your maternity leave (which is also "the 4th trimester"–birth to 3 months). You are still nurturing this growing life every bit as much as when you were pregnant, except now you've added crying, lactating, and never having free hands to the mix. That is your only project. We all wish we had known to expect nothing more from maternity leave than simple survival. Period.

ANNIE T., ANGIE G., AND SARITA C.

New Dads

> *Some people—dads, yes, but moms, too— can't (and don't) live at a fever pitch of emotion for more than a couple hours, tops. It's just too draining on them.*

Some new moms are surprised, disappointed or even downright ticked when their husbands or partners, now new dads, spend as much time "screen-sucking" (a.k.a., messing around with their Whatevers) as they do paying attention to their recovering wives and new babies.

This can be annoying, especially if you've seen other dads go absolutely bananas over their new babies, or heard stories about how "wonderful and thoughtful so-and-so was after I delivered—he brought me food, flowers and jumped up every time the baby made a sound. He didn't want to put her down for a second!" Or worse still, are reading from your hospital bed some incredibly heartfelt confession of gratitude and wonderment from a brand new dad on Facebook, as you watch your husband/partner play Candy Crush on his hand-held for the five millionth time.

Again, it's all about expectations. Some people— dads, yes, but moms, too—can't sustain such intense emotions for more than a couple of hours, tops. It's too draining. It could be that your husband/partner is so overwhelmed with the enormity of birth and fatherhood that he needs some time to himself to recharge. Playing a mindless game, texting with a friend, or watching sports on TV—having no idea the noise is driving you crazy—may be just what he needs to get his balance back after the emotions of the last few days.

Relationships are built moment by moment over days, weeks, and years. New moms need not interpret new dads' lack of utter fascination with their babies (and, let's be honest, their wives) as disinterest. He just may need time and space to regroup.

One more thing, not everyone is a "baby person." Many moms envision certain reactions from their babies' dads that may or may not occur. This unfulfilled expectation can be disappointing and hurtful. In Group, we talk sometimes about noticing the good that *is* happening, rather than what is *not* happening, and appreciating the unique positives each parent brings to the family.

More On New Dads

Now that you're home, this is where the rubber meets the road. Habits and practices will start to get set, and while a lot of moms feel the need to "protect" their partners from the insanity of newborn care, or feel inexplicably impatient with them for not "doing things right," getting Dad involved early and often is a huge bonus for everyone.

The more Dad interacts with baby, the more his confidence grows, the more breaks you have, the better baby and dad's relationship becomes. This is especially valuable when toddlerhood hits and everyone's patience gets stretched. Many new moms say if they had it to do over again, they would have made more of an effort to let Dad in, let him try, and let him (within reason) fail. After months of parenting, these moms see it's okay for parents to make mistakes. That's how we learn.

Looking 8 Months Pregnant with a Newborn

Most women say they know in their minds it takes time to lose the baby weight, but abstract knowledge doesn't make us any less uncomfortable or impatient with ourselves. The truth is, it's often 9 months on and 9 months off—or more. Your body is still in shock, and recovering from pregnancy and birth, and it will be that way for a while. You just spent 9 months gestating a new human life, for heaven's sake, there is bound to be some fallout—a term that also may describe the condition of your hair and your boobs at this point.

Not to worry–there are *many moms who* are in the same boat as you right now. While many of them put pressure on themselves to get back to pre-baby shape ASAP, it doesn't necessarily make it happen that much faster. Feel free to put those jeans on the highest closet shelf, (or better yet, have your husband/partner hide them from you), and don't even entertain the thought of trying them on until *at least* 6 months postpartum, and more like 9 to 12 months, for many.

The ugly truth is post-birth physical recovery takes time and can be frustrating. For some women, the whole experience took a toll on their self-esteem and enjoyment of early motherhood, and wish someone had told them they would still look pregnant long after they delivered. One mom said if she had it to do over again she would:

> *Keep a better sense of humor about what a train wreck a woman's body can be for a while after delivery. It isn't going to last forever, and breastfeeding alone burns a ton of calories. You just may not see the effects for several months because your body is adjusting to the new role of being a non-pregnant food source. I should have cut myself some slack, for God's sake. I mean, it's one year out of my whole life.*
>
> MARITA D.

Speaking for myself, quite honestly, I always hate how I look in the first 3 months postpartum, as I am not one of those women who "snaps back." I don't even like to take any pictures as a family during that time because *they* all look so cute, whereas I look fresh from Three Mile Island.

If it takes you more time to resemble yourself–body, hair, skin, coherence–than it seems to take others, you are not alone. It may take longer than you expected/hoped, but it'll happen. One thing to bear in mind, however, is that things may not be exactly where you left them, so to speak, as gravity begin to take its toll. As one mom said, "I'm not sure what's become of my tush, but my collar bone has never looked better."

Stitches, Coughing, and Laughing

With every cough I became more afraid that I was going to split my stitches and end up right back in the hospital like a stuck pig. I was totally freaking out.

INIRA V.

If you end up with stitches, whether across your belly, or "framing the old hoo-haw," as one second-time mom eloquently put it, coughing and laughing in the first week post-birth is going to hurt. With all the advice, papers, and general harassment so many new moms endure upon discharge and via the Internet, a critical mass of women have remarked that they wish someone had warned them before going home that any sneezing, laughing, and/or especially coughing with their new stitches would be not only painful, but a bit terrifying. Why terrifying? Here's what new mom Inira said:

I picked up some kind of bizarre virus or something in the hospital, and within 48 hours after discharge I started to cough uncontrollably for a few minutes every hour or so. It was awful on so many levels— trying to keep baby latched on, worrying that I'm passing on some mystery illness, and then feeling like I'm splitting my stitches from my episiotomy every time I had to cough, which I could not stop doing!

Every time the coughing spells came up, the stress on my stitches hurt so much I teared up. I was totally terrified that I was going to split my stitches and end up back in the hospital bleeding like a stuck pig, and I wouldn't be able to nurse my baby because I knew if I was admitted as an adult patient, they wouldn't allow me to keep a minor in my room, nor would they admit him as a pediatric patient. I was totally freaking out.

Finally, a friend of mine who happened to be over saw the kind of pain I was in. She had me sit on a towel, and pull it up between my legs whenever the coughing came on to keep pressure on the stitches. It did help some, as did her reassurances, but I was still so upset. It was painful and it was scary, and **no one said anything about it upon discharge.**

It only makes sense to me to tell postpartum patients, "If you have perineal stitches, sit on a towel and pull up (in other words, apply pressure) if you have to sneeze or cough (or laugh, though you may not be laughing about jack at this stage), and if you have abdominal stitches, hug a pillow or something to your lower belly. It will help." New moms need some instructions on how to cope with and care for their stitches. I was just lucky I had a friend over. A lot of women don't have anyone to help them through the post-birth stuff.

INIRA V.

More on Breastfeeding

Breastfeeding was way more frustrating than I ever thought it would be. Thank God for a good lactation consultant. I was ready to give up as a complete failure the 2nd night home when I just couldn't get him to eat, and all he would do is scream until he was hoarse. He finally started latching without a breast shield, but man, my nipples hurt.

DIANA B.

You're now probably somewhere between Day 3 and 23 of Breastfeeding, and you may be finding that it takes a while to get the hang of it. That's not the whole truth. You may be finding it's so painful you could die. Your baby may be latching on fine, and you're starting to produce milk, but you are so engorged you feel like your breasts are going to explode, and latching on hurts like no stinking book ever expressed. If you are still engorged, take steps immediately to alleviate it as it can drop your milk supply. Engorgement is not caused by milk in your breasts, but by other fluids. You need to bring that inflammation down using ibuprofen, cool compresses, and reverse pressure softening. Many mothers also find relief from putting cool cabbage leaves around their breasts.

If it hurts to latch, go see a lactation consultant or volunteer breastfeeding counselor. Chances are that with some slight adjustment, breastfeeding can be made much more comfortable. If breast-feeding hurts, get help. Don't just try to tough it out.

It's not uncommon during this stage of breast-feeding adjustment for moms to sometimes feel scared or upset when baby starts crying to be fed. Moms know they have to get baby on the breast again. In fact, one mother said:

> *When my husband asked what it feels like when the baby latches on, I politely suggested he go fetch a vice grip from his tool box and affix it to his &$#*. It actually may have been more hostile than polite, come to think of it, but he didn't ask again, and he was Johnny-on-the-spot with the Lanolin after that. "What does it feel like?" Do you really want to know?*
> *Natalie K.*

For the first 3 to 5 days postpartum, it may seem like nothing is happening breastfeeding-wise, but most moms feel their milk becomes more abundant somewhere around Day 5. Consider taking a bath towel to bed with you the first few weeks. Often your milk comes in and leaks all over you the moment, or moment before, baby cries out. No joke.

It can take a while to get the hang of breastfeeding, but it gets easier It may actually feel relaxing. You may feel the needle-like prickles of your milk coming in and letting down which some women find strange, but the latching will likely be nothing.

If breastfeeding hurts and/or you feel a lump in your breast, you could have a clogged duct or mastitis. Mastitis is a breast infection and is marked by a high fever, red streaking, and/or a hot spot(s) on the breast. This is serious and nothing to mess around with—so call your doctor's office as soon as possible. If it is mastitis, you will need a prescription for an antibiotic to recover. You should start feeling better about 12 hours after the first dose, but in the meantime it's like you've been hit by a train, so you'll want to start taking it ASAP.

Still Bleeding

Yep, you will be bleeding for up to a month following birth, though hopefully you have downgraded (or upgraded, depending on your perspective) from the crazy cheesecloth/mattress day to XL dollar bin underwear and super plus maximum strength maxis. But nonetheless, you are still bleeding. After not having your period for 9 months, you may find this a total pain in the neck. Or lower. Many women are shocked at how heavily they bleed, and for how long. Personally, I felt disgusting, but finding time to take a shower was, well, as I mentioned earlier, I flunked vertical hydrotherapy my first time around with motherhood, but I am now wiser. And more fragrant.

"Sleep When the Baby Sleeps"

Feel free to strangle anyone who suggests this. Seriously, it's a good idea in theory, and some can do it, but if you have other children at home, or you just can't fall asleep on cue, you don't have to stress yourself out. Instead, you can use the time to do something relaxing for yourself: take a shower, eat a meal in peace, "de-pile" the house, visit us at www.facebook.com/postpartumsupportflorida www.postpartumflorida.org, www.postpartum.net, or, as my aunt says, "Sit in a corner and drool."

Seriously, though, while it is unreasonable and downright annoying to feel pressured to sleep every time the baby sleeps, (WARNING: Advice pending) *protecting your sleep is of the utmost importance. Without sleep you will not feel well (read, "Crazy").* In fact, eventually you will get so used to being sleep-deprived, you won't even know you are exhausted. That's when things can get really messed up. *Consistently having trouble sleeping, even when the baby sleeps,* or staying awake between night feedings to write thank you notes or Christmas cards, *are red flags of potential Postpartum Distress.*

The one best thing you can do to support your physical and mental health is to *protect your sleep...* Now, hold on... before you get annoyed at me for saying that, believe me, I get it. I did not sleep more than one or two hours at a time after my first and fourth babies were born for months, and it nearly sent me around the bend. Getting sleep while caring for a newborn can be **extremely** challenging. That's why everyone says "sleep when the baby sleeps," right? Uh-huh.

Yet, for some women this strategy just intensifies their already deepening sense of confinement. If they sleep when their babies sleep, they never have any time alone to regroup, listen to silence, or simply concentrate. For that matter, if mom drops everything to sleep, who's going to do the laundry, pay the bills, and do the shopping? And when does a person eat, shower, or go to the bathroom? What if mom has older children to care for? Or has to go back to work outside the home? I don't know, Mama. I wish I had some satisfying answers.

It's not right or healthy that so many women have to shoulder so much alone. Still, the truth is *you are recovering from growing and pushing another human being out of your body, whom you now are caring for around the clock. Please consider grabbing sleep anytime you can, and do not feel guilty about it. It's just a few weeks or months out of your whole life.* If it helps, you can reframe the issue and imagine you are recovering from a major operation, or the flu, and you have to sleep to get your strength back.

Incidentally, I don't know why more physicians don't tell their postpartum patients to sleep as much as possible in the first 3 months post-birth. In many other cultures, postpartum mothers aren't even allowed out of bed for weeks or months. Clearly, other societies recognize that sleep isn't a bonus. It's as vital to wellness as nutrition and breathing, and we need to do better giving our new moms permission and encouragement to *prioritize and protect their sleep in the postpartum period.*

If you are not able to sleep, please reach out to www.postpartumflorida.org or www.postpartum.net for the resources you need so you can get some rest and prevent things from going downhill fast.

More on Older Children, Visitors, and Feeling Judged.

> *This is your recovery from birth. You have permission to do what you need to in order to take care of yourself so you are well and able to care of your baby. And if that means no visitors, then by all means, no visitors, no questions asked.*

It may come as a really crummy surprise to you that all the people you thought you'd be excited to share this beautiful experience with are not what the doctor ordered. At. All. Whether it's your children, your friends, your family or even your partner, you may feel like being left, in one mother's frank description, "the eff alone" with your baby, or even just "the eff alone" period.

When you consider all you've experienced throughout pregnancy, labor, delivery, and early postpartum, not to mention the conception period (as that can bring its own stresses for many couples), you may need, as the same mom said, "Some Goddamn space!" You can likely gather the raw, honest perspective she generously offered me, and she makes a powerful point–personal space is key to recharging and regaining some energy and balance following birth.

Some moms wish someone had told them they might *not* want to have a bunch of people around soon after birth (as in, a couple months), and if they change their minds about having visitors, whether at home or at the hospital, *that is okay*. In fact, this is your recovery from birth, and you have license do whatever you need to do to take care of *you,* so you are well and able to take care of your baby.

Many women have shared how guilty and conflicted they tend to feel about wanting or not wanting to spend time with their older children after a new baby comes. On one hand, a mom may be anxious to "put in some quality time" with her older children after being away in the hospital for a couple days (or more), but after taking the big kids to the science museum or the zoo, mom may feel completely exhausted, irritable, and frustrated that she couldn't make the outing work "the way it used to."

> *Anyone going from one to two kids, take note—there is a big adjustment period that is not so much on the kids' part, and it can really sucker punch you.*
>
> ANGIE G.

For some moms, it's difficult to face how the addition of a new baby will change what was a fairly settled family dynamic. A dynamic that may not have been perfect, but was familiar, comfortable, and (somewhat) predictable. When baby comes home, it may feel as if everything is up in the air. Not only is mom getting to know her new baby, she may also be feeling hyper-sensitive to all her children's (and her partner's) growing pains. This adjustment process can feel overwhelming and extremely stressful.

If you have had it up to your eyes with the caravan of well-meaning (or not so well-meaning) people traipsing through your home or hospital room, you are not being "difficult," "controlling," or "selfish." You are being honest with yourself, which is actually quite admirable, and an increasingly lost art.

Being honest about your needs during your postpartum adjustment is critical to your and your baby's wellness. This is where the "listening to your inner self" we talked about earlier comes into play. Being honest about one's needs can be difficult for some women and feel contrary to their self-sufficient personalities. Sometimes needing *anything* from *anyone* makes a woman feel selfish, demanding, or terribly vulnerable. Still, the adjustment to motherhood can be a good time to experiment with letting one's guard down a little and allowing more support from others. Yet opening ourselves up to other people is complicated, isn't it?

The presence of others can breed unintentional pressure, too. New moms frequently feel the watchful, critical eyes of others–their partners, their mothers, their in-laws (!), and even their friends–judging them in the early days (or years) of motherhood. This pressure can add to a woman's postpartum stress. The truth is, when people judge you, it's more about them than it is about you. Most people organize the information they take in into boxes of approval and disapproval (a.k.a., making judgments) because they are psychologically hard-wired to do so, not because they are necessarily trying to drive you crazy — even though it may have that net effect.

Everyone–including those who deeply love you–will make judgments and draw nonsensical conclusions about your parenting choices. Their judgments do not mean you're doing anything wrong, nor is it anything you can control. Most important, it's powerful only if you give it power. It *is* within your control to *refuse* to give other people's judgments any power over you.

It's okay to let go of worrying about what others think of you, your parenting decisions, and your style of hospitality in the postpartum period (or entirely, but that's another book). Let go, and let go, and let go. You have permission to let go of self-conscious anxiety every time it arises. Let it go. Breathe it out. Move on. The postpartum period is so intense, you have every right to change your feelings about having visitors and family (and their remarks) at any time, and that's understandable to any reasonable person. (By the way, if you ever come across a reasonable person, please let me know).

Now, to be fair, getting the visitors to go away will not be an issue for everyone. There are women for whom visitors will be a highlight, and sharing the birth, the coming home and/or the early days of newbornhood with friends and family will be extremely important. She will want those who matter most to her to visit, meet her new baby, and be present for a portion of her experience. In fact, she will likely be offended if her friends and family do *not* come over, spend time with her, and meet her new baby. One mother of almost five said this about postpartum visitors:

> *Time and time again, friends and family have wanted to come as soon as we get*

home, or even in the hospital. I get it—it's fun to come visit your friend and her newborn in the hospital, largely because when it's you in the hospital, there's nothing the least bit enjoyable about it (Please see Chapter 4: Older Siblings and Visitors). Similarly, I know it's "fun" to see a brand-new little baby that's just come home. That said, this time I'm saying "No" to visitors for at least the first 2 weeks. This little guy will have plenty of time to get to know everyone, and I can't wait to introduce him when I don't feel like absolute garbage.

When I had my fourth child, the day I got home, two very excited, well-meaning friends came to bring meals and "meet the baby" because, of course, it's really special to see a brand-new baby. However, God bless them, they stayed for almost an hour! AN HOUR!!! I still could barely sit down at that point, was trying to get my daughter to latch, was completely exhausted from not sleeping more than 3 hours at a time for nearly 9 months, felt self-conscious that my older children were climbing the walls, and was still so nauseated from the after pains that I could hardly focus on the words they were saying, much less respond appropriately.

Honestly, 10 minutes would have been okay, and up to 20 could have been somewhat permissible, but an hour???? I still have no real clue what occurred during that visit, but I'm not going to tempt fate again, even if I have to make something up. I'm fully prepared to say I contracted rotavirus in the hospital and don't want to infect them. "Love you dearly—catch up with you in 2 weeks (at least!)."

MARILYN T.

Another experienced mom had this advice/strategy for the visitor dilemma.

When it comes to visitors at home, your willing scapegoat is your pediatrician. When everyone and their brother wants to manhandle your days-old baby, feel free to kick everyone out and say, "Baby's doc says no visitors for two weeks/for x days after vaccines, etc." The first part is true. The rest of it just maintains your sanity and keeps people and their germy kids away!

TRACEY B.

Nutrition

At some point in the first month postpartum, you realize you don't have two hands to do things anymore. You mostly don't even have one. Now those one-handed, high-protein, high-fat snacks from Chapter One really come in handy. Think nuts (chocolate covered, naturally), cheese sticks, shelled hard-boiled eggs, and dry breakfast cereal. Whether you are breastfeeding or not, your body needs to recover.

The food/nutrition thing can get especially complicated, and bring on guilt and negative thoughts because quick sugar might be one of the only things that keeps you going and/or is a source of enjoyment right now. After the birth of my third child, I kept an open bag of chocolate chips on the kitchen counter from the third week to probably the fourth month postpartum. I figured, "If this is the worst the vices get, we're doing fine."

"Bumpy Start"/Sensitive Babies

The mom of a more sensitive newborn often feels embarrassed or apologetic that her baby is having more of a bumpy start, as well as guilty that she's not enjoying her baby as much as she expected to or as much as other new moms seem to be enjoying their babies.

This is tough stuff for everyone: tough to recover, tough to bond, tough to communicate with your partner, and maybe tough to feel like things will ever get better. One mom of a "bumpy start" baby said:

We tried every frickin' thing with Baby L— swing, swaddle, shush, gas drops, Reglan, in case he had reflux, you name it. He's just intense, and gets so screamy when he's tired, which doesn't help him fall asleep. During his first 2 months, I spent hours every night sitting on a stability ball, bouncing him. It was the only thing that would calm him. I still use it when he gets really squirrelly tired.

He started responding to a bouncy seat with a nice, peppy bounce so Daddy could get in on the baby-soothing action. The little guy had so much trouble figuring out when he wanted to sleep. Things got better, but it took a long time to get to a good place, for his happiness and ours.

ANGIE G.

"Bumpy start" babies present a unique degree of postpartum stress. In fact, having a bumpy start baby immediately puts mom (and dad) at the head of the line for postpartum support. The mom of a bumpy start baby often feels embarrassed, or apologetic, that her baby is more sensitive at this stage, and that (of course) she's not enjoying her baby as much as she expected to, and/or other new mothers seem to be enjoying their babies, and as a consequence may be less likely to reach out for post-partum support. Such a shame, as the wonderful parents of bumpy start babies often need support the most! A normal response, but as one mom said:

> *I wish someone had told me to just tell the truth about how I felt. Trying to hide my ambivalent feelings about my high-need newborn daughter in her first very, very rocky 8 weeks made my transition and caring for her exponentially more stressful. Once she started sleeping a few hours at a time, and we got through the worst of it, we started to bond for real, and it made all the pretending seem really stupid. It was what it was, and that's life. We went through some serious crap together, and even though I still can't really face what happened in those first 2 months, if I had to do it again, it would have been better for me to be honest about what was happening so I could work through it and get some help.*
>
> NATALIE K.

One mom remembered her days with her easily over-stimulated/sensitive baby very well, and recalled what eventually helped things improve:

> *I finally realized he didn't like being a baby. Once he could roll over, then crawl and walk, we had so much fun together. When we were both cranky, I did a lot of "fake it 'til you make it." I smiled at him whether I*

felt like it or not, and it helped both of us feel better.

I feel for moms of intense, sensitive babies that don't want to be lying in one spot, and always want to be bounced/held/looking around—it can be exhausting. You'll have such fun together when he can be more independent. What a fantastic little person you have in your arms. Being a baby just isn't his (or her) style.

GRACIE W.

Going Bald and Other Signs of Hagdom

Many of the pregnancy and "First Year" books talk casually about "hormone changes," and "your body adjusting to breastfeeding/not being pregnant," but what many new mothers wish someone had told them is that you may sort of go bald, and generally look like a hag for a while after you give birth. This does not happen to everyone, which makes spreading the word all the more vital.

Frequently new moms lament that they drag themselves, engorged and balding, to a new-moms group, only to find every other mom there looks amazing! *Amazing!!* Like, going-out-with-full-hair-and-make-up-amazing. Baffled, the haggish moms observe these perfected individuals with disbelief. "How can she look so great? I have one contact in, and I don't think I even brushed my teeth!" Following their initial shock, these half-blind, gum-chewing moms wonder then turns to discomfort and self-consciousness. "Why can't I pull myself together? She doesn't look like her hair is coming out in clumps and... Yes, yes... those are buttons on her jeans, dammit, buttons! I'm still muffin-topping over my maternity pants!"

(Sigh)... Postpartum recovery–it's not pretty, but you *always* are, Mama, and that's a fact. Even when you don't feel like it. You are doing the hardest job there is–caring for a new human being, and that alone makes you divine, marvelous, and extraordinary (plus all your other regular awesomeness, of course). As Dorothy of *The Golden Girls* once wisely said, "It's not easy being a mother. If it were, fathers would do it."

Bottom line, if you don't look at all like yourself for a while–as in "months"–after you deliver, you may kind of hate it, but it is 100% normal. I don't know how anyone could possibly **NOT** feel like the walking dead after growing, carrying, and pushing a brand new person out of her own body, and then becoming her round-the-clock food source/supplier, for heaven's sake. Please know this–a lot of stuff goes down in the first 12 months post-birth, but you will find your spring again. Just be aware, however, that like pregnancy it's a process of months, not days.

For what it's worth, we are allowed to dial down our personal expectations and let it ride through the first year. There is no perfect wife, mother, or woman. You *are* amazing exactly as you are, and you will meet whatever long-term goals you have for yourself. Moreover, we have no idea what's going on in the lives of these alleged "perfect-looking people." It's a cliché, but you really can't judge a book by its cover, and what's more, a little hagdom keeps us humble. As one mom put it:

I looked like death warmed-over for at least 2 months after my son was born, and honestly, it took longer for everything to come back online with each subsequent child. However, I now accept this about myself. I can take the time to put on concealer and perfume, and at least re-do my ponytail, but sometimes I just don't give a rat's a**, and that's my choice.

At first, I thought if I didn't look like my pre-pregnant self on the same schedule as other new moms it meant I was "behind" or wouldn't get there, but after going through the cycle a few times, I know that's not true. It just takes some of us a little longer. I'd rather have 15 more minutes of sleep or stillness than get up and do my hair and make-up to go somewhere, and get spit-up, poop, or breastmilk on myself. I'll start caring again next year. That's how I feel and I'm good with it.

CHRISTINA C.

The one thing is—it's overused, but true—put on your own oxygen mask first and don't feel one bit guilty about it. As one mom said:

> *Keep up with self-care—fluids, vitamins, nutrition, teeth brushing, etc. Our Pedi said he can always tell the mother is having a hard time when she brings in an adorable, well-dressed, glowing little cutie, and mom looks like she's been in a war zone. Shows that she's putting herself way last and is headed for possible burn-out.*
>
> JANE P.

It's very healthy to let things go. Sometimes we have to let things go *repeatedly*, such as disappointment over a birth experience, or hurt that husband doesn't "get it," multiple times a day because holding on to hurt and disappointment only stresses us out, limits us and holds us back. But completely letting *yourself* go, a.k.a., not taking care of yourself, is not going to work. Many new mothers say they wish they'd known it was okay to do things to take care of themselves, and it doesn't mean they're being selfish, so here goes, ahem. "It is okay to do things for yourself. That is being smart, NOT being selfish!" Any questions?

Missing Being Pregnant

I wish we cared as much about the Post-partum Mom as we seem to be fascinated by the Pregnant Mom-to-Be. I didn't really need doors opened for me when I was pregnant, but juggling a toddler, a stroller, three bags, and a hungry newborn? Yep, now would be a great time to hold open that door.

NATALIE K.

Missing being pregnant is normal, and a lot of women feel it, even if they don't admit it. In our Postpartum Support Group, some women have said they were surprised they missed being pregnant, especially those who were sick through most of their pregnancy, were on bed rest, or had other complications. Why do they miss being pregnant? As one second-time mother said:

You feel so special when you're pregnant. People ask you how you're doing, once your belly pops it looks so cute (for a while), and, of course, feeling the baby move is just the best. After I gave birth, I just felt so empty. I looked at my floppy stomach in the mirror, and looked and felt awful. I missed feeling my son against me. I wore him in the sling so I could feel him. It helped a little. It was hard.

Then once baby comes, instead of being Super Pregnant Lady, I'm just another woman with a crying baby trying to nurse in a checkout line. I wish we cared as much about the Post-partum Mom as we seem to be fascinated by the Pregnant Mom-to-Be. I didn't really need doors opened for me when I was pregnant, but juggling a toddler, a stroller, three bags, and a hungry newborn? Yep, now would be a great time to hold open that door

NATALIE K.

What You Need to Recharge

Many, many new moms feel overwhelmed and powerless at times (or for some, all the time) as they adjust to motherhood. Yet, it seems every magazine article on postpartum wellness says the same thing: exercise, eat leafy greens, go on a date night. Give me a break. The standard coffee table recipe for postpartum wellness falls far short of what actual mothers need. Mothers are still women–individual and unique, not some Stepford focus group, and shoving all moms into lockstep on how to (properly) relax. Guess what? Not relaxing!

Some women need to order their environment to get their heads straight. Others need time alone to reflect and organize their *inner* worlds/inner selves so they can feel a sense of control and balance. Still other moms may feel trapped being at home so much in the first few months, and while many mamas are devoted to breastfeeding and won't give it up, some may feel confined by a rigid nursing schedule, lonely without friendly adults to laugh with, and generally, as one mom put it, "stuck." (Please visit www.post-partumflorida.org and click on "Personality and PPD" and "Our PPD Study" for more information on the impact of personality differences in the post-partum period).

Every mother (really, every person) needs something specific to emotionally recharge, especially under stressful circumstances. Some crave privacy, quiet, and limited interruptions. Others ache for freedom, connection, and variety. In order for a new mom to recover, care for baby, and healthfully adjust to the demands of motherhood, her individual needs have to be recognized, respected, and responded to. I want to emphasize that needing to relax and regroup has nothing to do with a mother's love for her baby. Everyone needs time and space to recharge in her own way. *Everyone.*

It's super-convenient if someone recharges by baking a thousand chicken breasts to freeze, or thoroughly scrubbing a highchair and car seat, or making matching handcrafted outfits for every occasion, but those preferences don't make that person a *better* mother. It just makes her transition to motherhood a little smoother. How lucky to overlap your current responsibilities with your personal interests. Other moms may dread cleaning and cooking, and can't even thread a needle, but have fascinating talents and interests that just don't happen to coincide with the common demands of newborn care and early motherhood.

Every mom is specific and necessary, and when there is little to no space for her best features and qualities to be expressed in the postpartum period, she may feel self-conscious, and doubt her abilities as a mom. The trick to getting through the "heaviness" of postpartum adjustment is to carve out tiny spaces within your changing world to stay tethered to your inner self as you find your new rhythm.

It's not the whole enchilada of who you are, and the bridge from pre-baby-you to mother-you may be bumpy, but the postpartum year is the boot camp of motherhood. It's tough, intense, and exhausting, but it is finite. It gets easier, and you will do it, and do it well. You may not enjoy it all the time, or feel comfortable with the changes that are happening to you—postpartum is much like adolescence that way—but you can carry your uniqueness forward into motherhood, find that new normal, and create your own original new you.

Beware of "Perfect" Mothers

"All that glitters is not gold," as my mother says, and any new mom who lassos you into a conversation about how well her baby is nursing, how fast she lost the weight, how long baby is sleeping through the night, how much big brother/sister just *adores* his/her baby, blah blah blah, is either compensating for something, and/or just took her fourth non-prescription antidepressant of the day.

Guess what? You do not have to be her friend. You do *NOT* have to give her your number to "get the babies together." She will only make you crazy. The quiet moms in the playgroup are harder to get to know amid all the crying, but much more stable, real, and worth knowing. Many new moms say they wish they'd known you don't have to try to become close friends with any and all new moms you meet. "Just 'cause you both have babies doesn't mean you're going to besties," one first-time mom said.

It's sort of like going to camp or college, and trying to make friends. You end up talking to/ hanging around with the people you're sitting with on the first day. Then, after a few weeks or months, you realize you actually don't feel that comfortable with them. You may choose to disentangle yourself from these friends, find new ones, and even go through the process of wondering, "What's wrong with me that I didn't click with them?"

Truth? There's nothing wrong with you at all. In fact, you're awesome! You're reading, reaching out, trying to make sense of all the postpartum craziness. ... Hell yeah, Mama, *you're rocking this!!* It's simply that making new "mom friends" is just like camp, college, and cafeterias. It takes time, and there are lots of women out there who you *will* truly click with. You just weren't sitting with them on the first day. If you keep going to different mom-and-baby gatherings, and keep being yourself (even if that person seems to be constantly changing as you find your "New Normal"), you will meet women you really like and develop a lifelong bond with them-- like a hostage situation.

Death, Grief, and Postpartum Stress

> *Frequently new mothers who are grieving the death of a loved one or a previous pregnancy or infant loss may find themselves shocked by the intensity of their grief, and so pressed by the needs of their new baby, as well as other children and responsibilities, they have little personal/ emotional space to grieve, and may struggle to manage their stress.*

Losing someone you love is a pain beyond words, and whether expected or unexpected, past or present, sometimes mothers are shaken when their babies' arrival triggers a new grieving period for a past loss. What's worse, it may be hard for others to accept that a mama who's felt the pain of pregnancy loss, stillbirth, infant or child death may need time to grieve in a new way. To many folks, this may look like "wallowing" or "living in the past" when "she has a baby now and *should* be happy!" Ugh! Wrong answer!

It's only natural to think about the ones you've loved and lost as you learn to love another; imagining the joys you dreamed of having beside a little one who's no longer with you as you build memories with a new sweetheart. Love, life, and death are about as complicated as it gets, and (newsflash), *mothers are capable of having more than one emotion at a time.* We can be mournful *and* grateful, overjoyed *and* overwhelmed all at once! Astonishing, isn't it? Enough "shoulding" all over ourselves.

Explaining it this way may help others understand. All the precious people a mother treasures are carefully kept in her heart. When her heart grows a new room for her new baby, the loves, dreams, and losses she's experienced may knock around against each other for a while until her heart settles down again. It's not about forgetting—a mother never forgets.It's about reordering our world, and learning to cope with grief in our new circumstances.

In addition to past losses, some of the moms in our support group suffered the loss of a loved one during their postpartum year. These moms were shocked to discover their stress and grief-coping responses were "wobblier" during the postpartum period than they would have been were they not caring for a vulnerable new baby. In fact, frequently new mothers who are grieving the death of a loved one find themselves overwhelmed by the intensity of their grief, and so pressed by the needs of their new baby, as well as other children and responsibilities, they have little personal/emotional space to grieve. This can make coping a challenge, and exaggerate post-birth stress.

If you, or someone you know, experiences a loss or a resurfacing of grief in the postpartum period, and are suffering, please know the key to coping can be as simple as *talking about it with someone you trust.* It may be difficult to find that person within your family if your family members are grieving, too, but there are places you can go for real, thoughtful support. Grief and loss groups can be a tremendous help, including online support through Facebook Groups and BabyCenter. I am so sorry for any loss you've suffered. Peer support in times of tragedy can be an incredibly powerful tool for healing. Please know you are not alone.

Your Inner Conversation

Many new mothers are caught off-guard by the doubt and worry they feel over even their earliest parenting decisions. The combination of the hormone changes, sleep deprivation, and physical and emotional exhaustion can trigger an inner monologue of worry and negativity. If unchecked, this negative self-talk can devolve into a self-destructive habit of anxiety and doubt that multiplies when you're already stretched to your maximum.

Ugh! Negative thoughts! They are a drag, and especially wily and destructive with new, isolated moms since conversing with a baby is a uniquely one-sided conversation. Negative thoughts wear convincing disguises, too—virtue, honor, selflessness, kindness, sympathy, achievement, pride, even martyrdom. These negative, critical thoughts can seem valid, like they're giving you good advice, but if the so-called "good advice" is riddled with those nasty "shoulds" we just discussed, "inner insults," and obscenities. Exhaustion has shut off your internal filter, and your mind is spinning free of gravity. It's not uncommon, but it sure is torture.

When negative thoughts start looping through your sleep-deprived, addled mind, you have the power to stop them, or at least slow them down. Every time one pops up, you have the power to replace it with an opposite, positive thought, even hundreds of times a day. Just because it popped into your unfiltered mind doesn't mean you need to take it in, try to understand it, or believe it.

We can choose which thoughts to concentrate on like we choose which foods to eat. Even in the overwhelming fatigue of the postpartum period, what we listen to and believe in our own minds is still our choice. We can speak to ourselves with kindness and patience. We can nourish ourselves with positive, encouraging thoughts. Instead of worrying, "I can't do this," we can tell ourselves, "I *can* do this. I AM doing this. I'm just not enjoying it yet." "I am a good mother. I don't have to be 'perfect' to be good. This is really hard, and it will get easier. I am working really, really hard, and doing a good job."

You can tell yourself good things over and over, hundreds of times a day. Positive thinking is free, and it definitely can't hurt, though during the exhausting postpartum period the required effort and concentration can be tough to muster. Yet, positive self-talk is a powerful tool, especially if you're game to make it a habit. It requires no membership fees, expensive starter kits, or outfits to squeeze into, no shipping costs, child care, or parts to clean. Nope, this wellness technique starts right in your rocking chair because feeling happier can begin with us accepting that we *already* approve of ourselves *exactly as we are.*

We are good, and can never be anything but good. We have the free will to do dumb things, but we, in truth, are *good. Good* mothers, *good* people, *good* daughters, and *good* partners. We can love ourselves exactly as we are because we are already so lovable. We just have to believe it. We exude good every day. Knowing it, and owning our awesomeness, can be the key to lifelong health and happiness. Why isn't this simple habit of positive self-talk more popular, revered, and taught to every new mama to share with her family? Easy. Because it's not a money-maker. There's no gadget to buy and throw away. No system to "sell." Just us, taking a stand against the inner bully.

Please know I struggled with talking nicely to myself *for years,* so I don't mean to say it's an easy switch, but for many people it really works. Personally, I started making the change after my fourth child to when Postpartum Anxiety came creeping. At Postpartum Florida we also use positive affirmation exercises in our Moms' Support Group, as well as our volunteer trainings, and I can honestly say I have been *amazed* by the personal breakthroughs some moms have made by committing to changing their inner conversation, and shutting that bully down.

Positive self-talk can turn things around, and, for some mamas, allow them to take their lives back. Quick heads-up—it takes about 6 weeks to switch your brain over from old "reflex" negative thoughts to new positive ones, and will require daily attention. So if you're having a hard time making the change for a while, it's okay. Those old inner bully grooves run deep, but if it's something you want to do, you'll get there. It's as easy as complimenting yourself on all the good you do every day, the exceptional gifts you bring to your family and community, and how amazing you are. And you are. Period.

It's so simple we sometimes forget. If we eat crud, we feel like crud, and if we ruminate on inner insults, criticism, and regret, our hearts and minds can feel defensive, bitter, and hopeless. Entertaining ongoing negative thoughts and guilt really *is* like allowing yourself to be bullied from the inside. You wouldn't want that kind of abuse for anyone you love, including the most important person in your family: *you*. You are too good for that garbage.

A Last Word About Breastfeeding

If you are breastfeeding, and your baby is 1 to 3 weeks old, you may be at the point where latching on has become incredibly painful. If it is, get help for it ASAP. It is not a normal part of breastfeeding. Don't wait until your nipples are shredded or you get an infection. If you are a few weeks in, you are in the home stretch. By one month postpartum, you'll be an expert at breastfeeding.

There are other warning signs of problems. Some moms I've known have shared that they experienced breastfeeding pain for weeks or even months that was shrugged off or dismissed by breastfeeding support counselors or select lactation consultants as "unexplainable," or due to the "low pain tolerance" of the mother. However, experienced IBCLCs state that breastfeeding pain is *not* normal and must be addressed immediately. If you are not getting the help or answers you need to alleviate your breastfeeding pain and correct the problem from your current lactation support person, *please reach out for a different professional and/or volunteer.* Or if you are too overwhelmed with newborn care and personal recovery, have your partner or family member/ friend investigate options and advocate for you.

Specifically, if you have a lump in your breast, cracking and/or bleeding nipples, or simply feel that something about the way breastfeeding is going with your baby just isn't right, you can reach out right away to your hospital's lactation consultant, call your local La Leche League, or find a breastfeeding support group in your community. Furthermore, if you have red streaking on your breast, one or more hot spots on your breast, or a high fever with chills you may have mastitis, and you need to call your provider right away.

There are many things that can help a difficult breastfeeding situation, and having nursed four babies for a total of four and a half years, I can honestly say I am so glad I was able to breast-feed my children for many reasons–the bonding, the nutrition, and my own physical recovery (the release of oxytocin during breastfeeding was about the only thing that relaxed me with my third child). So, if breastfeeding is a goal of yours, you do not need to feel discouraged by the fumbling of the first few weeks.

For some moms, however, breastfeeding is not possible, and if it doesn't work out as planned, it can be disappointing, stressful, and, for some moms, devastating. Especially if the mother has associated some (or all) of her success as a mother on her ability to breastfeed. In other situations, bottle-feeding may have been planned, but the process of "drying up," dealing with others' disapproval, and figuring out "how to bond with the bottle" can be a lot to manage. A first-time mother shared her struggle with breastfeeding, and how she transitioned to bottle-feeding in a positive way:

Not being able to breastfeed was one of the most difficult obstacles I had to overcome as a new mom. When I was pregnant, I had every intention to breastfeed, so much that I didn't even have any bottles before my daughter was born because I didn't think I would need them. All the childbirth education classes talk about how important the bonding is between mother and infant during breastfeeding, and I was so looking forward to that experience.

Towards the end of my pregnancy when the colostrum didn't come in I started to get a little worried, but my OB told me that was "normal," that it came later for some mothers, and not to worry because once the baby comes I would have plenty to feed her.

When my daughter was finally born and first placed on my chest there is no word to describe the emotions I was feeling. I immediately tried breastfeeding, but we were unsuccessful in the delivery room so the nurses told me to try again later. That this was normal to experience difficulty in the beginning. Time after time, I tried feeding her during my stay in the hospital, but it seemed I did not have any breast milk or colostrum yet.

Everyone kept telling me it was normal, to be patient, that it could take a week sometimes for milk to come in. I wanted to believe them, yet I was so nervous to bring her home because I didn't know how to feed her and I didn't want to give her a bottle. The disappointment I felt was overwhelming, I felt that I was already failing as a mother and I hadn't even brought her home yet. I couldn't stop thinking that I was doing something wrong, and I beat myself up over it for a long time.

At home the inability to breastfeed continued, and I got increasingly discouraged and frustrated. I had breastfeeding consultants come to my house. I went to breastfeeding support groups, online forums, I talked to my OB, my daughter's pediatrician, and everyone kept telling me to keep trying. But nothing was happening.

Going to support groups was also discouraging because everyone was whipping out their breasts to nourish their children and here I was whipping out some chemically made concoction. I felt like such a failure and that everyone was judging my formula-fed baby and me. I even put off feeding my wailing infant a time or two until I left the "support" groups to avoid embarrassment at not having the means to sustain her. Everyone kept saying, "Don't give up, don't give up, and keep trying." So I didn't give up.

I started pumping five to 10 times a day in an attempt to stimulate my milk, and barely got splatters in the bottle. I clearly remember sitting on my bed in the middle of the night crying and attempting to pump my empty breast while my husband sat feeding formula to our baby next to me. I decided shortly thereafter that the attempt to breastfeed had become such a stress that it was taking too much energy and time away from my daughter.

I stopped trying after about 3 months and started focusing on trying to bond with the bottle. I started talking to her while giving her the bottle, stroking her head, looking in her eyes, and I soon started to feel that bond everyone talks about when feeding your baby. When I think back on it now, I don't have any regrets. I know I did what I had to do, and my relationship with my beautiful daughter has never been affected by my inability to breastfeed.

REBECCA L.

Burping the Baby

This isn't really a baby care book, but please permit me to share with you one *extremely important baby-care tip* I wish someone had told *me*. *Burp the baby really, really well*, especially in the first 3 to 4 months. I was too timid to be diligent about it, and I'm certain *my oldest child would have slept better and stayed asleep longer if I had adequately burped him.*

You can ask your pediatrician and/or childbirth educator the best way to burp a baby. After four babies, I've found a firm pat on baby's lower back/bottom while doing a deep bounce (bend those knees!) with baby high on your chest/shoulder works well. Sometimes baby needs to burp two or three times in a row to get tummy relief, and if you feed baby and then put him/her in the car seat and s/he starts crying? Probably needs to burp. I can't say it enough... *burp the baby really well and every time* and you'll both feel better.

Sex. No, Seriously

I had a small 2ⁿᵈ-degree tear and that puppy didn't heal until 9 weeks postpartum. Separate from that, I had zero, and I mean ZERO, libido for damn close to 6 months. Thankfully, my husband is a patient man.

ANGIE G.

Another lovely postpartum surprise for new moms (and dads): postpartum hormones are designed to get you focused on taking care of the baby you have, not having another one. If your libido tanks in every possible way in the weeks (and months) after birth, please know it's normal and you're not the only one. Aren't surprises fun?

I love what a friend and mother of three had to say about postpartum sex (or lack thereof):

> *The last thing on earth you will want with lochia oozing from your vag, milk shooting out your nipples, and a critter constantly hanging on you, is to get jiggy with The Mister. Your OB is your willing scapegoat. He/she will tell you "no nookie til the first postpartum visit," which won't be for at least 6 weeks (maybe 8). Feel free to tell the Spousal after that appointment that OB says you need to heal for another 2 weeks. It happens especially with episiotomies and tears.*
>
> TRACEY B.

The lack of remotely satisfying intimacy (or any intimacy) in the postpartum period can further strain the relationship of two already thoroughly exhausted people (or one thoroughly exhausted person, and one person on the first person's sh*t list). But it seems to be worse if you and your partner think you are the only ones. Feel free to grab the man for this page. I'll wait. Okay, ready? Ahem...

YOU ARE NOT THE ONLY ONES NOT HAVING SEX LIKE YOU USED TO. YOU ARE RIGHT IN THE DRY-SPELL MAINSTREAM. If both people (okay, usually the guy) can be patient, helpful, and understanding, things will start heating up again a lot faster than if he's frumping and moping around, basically needing as much attention as another child.

Here's a newsflash, dads:

FRUMPY + MOPEY + NEEDY = NOT SEXY

Now check this out:

COMPLIMENTS + HOUSEWORK + BABY CARE = SEXY

I understand this formula is the higher math of monogamy, but I believe you fellas can handle it. Study, review, make flashcards if you must, but this is the one thing new dads wish someone had told *them*. You don't want to end up so far out in the cold that you see on the back of your wife's pajamas, "Closed for Business–please call again. Next Year."

Vacations, Weekends, and Holidays

Oy! There's no easy way to break this to you, so I'm just going to say it flat out: Moms work harder on vacations, evenings, weekends, and holidays than they do any other time of the year. Most new mothers don't necessarily feel this shift right out of the blocks, but often somewhere around month 4 to 6 postpartum, you may realize you and baby have achieved something resembling a "routine" of feeding and sleeping, and any shift in that routine can unravel a precise and treasured formula for (everyone's) sleep. This can make travel difficult.

What used to be fun and spontaneous adventures, or even just well-planned long weekends pre-baby, are now a juggling act of what you (and/or you partner) *want* to do against what you feel you *need* to do for your baby's routine. Frequently, new moms feel a bit disappointed that "going away" with baby feels a little like, as one mom said, "Throwing yourself into a crackling fire pit just to see what happens. You know it won't be good, but you're just stupid enough to try."

This won't be every mother's perspective, of course, but if you used to enjoy vacations, weekends, and holidays as special times of fun, relaxation, and time to recharge with your partner, and especially enjoyed being part of holidays, but not really "taking charge" of the holiday preparation and execution, well, times are changing. Many moms work harder during these "down times" than any other time of the day or the year. And all those wonderful holiday memories that you cherished and looked forward to creating for and/or sharing with your family. Who made all that possible? Yes, indeed, likely someone's *mother,* and she worked her tail off to do it. This may be a good time to call her and say thanks. I have some laundry to do anyway. Meet you back in 10.

"I Can't Stand My Husband"

Ah yes, that old chestnut. If I had a dime for every time a new mom has said (or thought) the above, this book would come with a bonus tennis bracelet just to cheer you up. Truly, despising one's husband is such a running theme in our Postpartum/Mothers of Little Ones Support Group, I don't even know where to begin. I tend to tread lightly on this topic because as much as women feel irritated with their partners, they are protective of them, too, and they are not eager to bad-mouth them only to wind up the subject of gossip or pity. That said, every mom needs to vent and know she's not alone in her feelings and struggles. Many, if not most, new moms go through periods of thinking their husbands/ partners are total idiots. I don't know if this is yet another iteration of nature's birth-control methods, but I do know if you've ever felt this way, you are definitely *not* alone!

To be fair, postpartum is really tough on dads, too. They have no idea what's happening to their partners emotionally and physically, and they can't fix it, so they often cope by shutting down. Women, on the other hand, tend to equate love with understanding, i.e., "If you loved me, you'd try to understand me." In a perfect world, that would be true, but understanding one's wife in the postpartum phase can be a tall order for a man. Can any man really relate to the female perinatal experience? Even with the best of intentions? I don't think so.

Here's what he may be able to do. He can help out with tasks and show love and concern in his own way. That said, I have also observed that most men cannot fully understand the complexity of their wives' feelings and changes in the postpartum period, especially since *exhaustion exaggerates emotions*. Remember when we were younger? The differences between teenage boys and teenage girls? Straightforward v. Complex? Once again this dichotomy rears its ugly head.

For the record, I am not trying to insult anyone. Many men have a beautiful capacity to be thoughtful, loving, and have deep feelings, but postpartum is super-intense emotional stuff no matter who you are. For a new dad, just trying to keep up with his wife's deep feelings (and how quickly they change) is often challenging, confusing, and frustrating. This is why *women truly need other women as they recover from birth and adjust to motherhood.*

Still, it's really lousy to despise the very person you, up until recently, were quite fond of, and attempt to adjust to parenthood amid a fog of tension. The stress of feeling misunderstood and irritated that your partner "just doesn't get it," combined with needing him *and* hating him all at once, can make a new mom feel more alone and unsupported than ever.

The good news is women actually have a lot of power to dispel family tension by taking charge of situations and working the old "fake it 'til you make it." If the feelings of conflict are really getting you down, and you can't yet fix how you feel on the inside (postpartum adjustment takes time), sometimes it works to start on the outside. By choosing to change some of our external behaviors, we can get things moving in a better direction.

Some new moms were glad to know they don't have to sort out their every feeling with their husbands, that parsing through each frustration doesn't necessarily solve anything or improve the relationship, and that *lots of couples are going through the exact same thing*. These ladies said they felt empowered knowing they could pick and choose what to share with whom, they could draw some boundaries around themselves, and keep certain things within their circle of women.

Please know, I'm not advocating concealing your true feelings, or hiding anything about you or your wellness from your partner. These are simply a few ways to replace old, conflict-producing habits that aren't working with new, different habits when the monotony of daily life in early parenthood starts to grind on both of you, and small things mushroom into huge fights.

Instead of ratcheting through the insanity of life as the stay-at-home-mom of little ones (i.e., how many times you've cleaned the kitchen today, how much poop you've wiped off assorted living beings, and how many bodily fluids you've been sprayed with), some of our Group moms made the deliberate choice to smile at their partners (whether they felt like it or not) when they first saw them. They actually practiced (it takes practice–these are new habits!) keeping their faces relaxed and open (eyebrows up), and a relaxed, even tone of voice. Oh, and saying, "Sweetheart" through gritted teeth unfortunately doesn't count. After all, it isn't what you say, it's how you say it, right?

You may be staring at this book right now thinking, "Are you kidding me? *Smile* at him? After the day I've had and the way he acts? He doesn't deserve it!" Hey, I totally get it. This isn't what you *should* do. It's what you *could* do. It all may sound disingenuous, or just plain ridiculous. If you hate it, don't do it. But for some moms, changing their external behaviors helped improve everyone's moods, and broke the cycle of exhausted cynicism that's so common in early parenting.

Sometimes women feel pressure to "make everyone happy" before they let themselves be happy, and then are pretty ticked when no one appreciates their efforts. And when Mom's not happy, no one's happy. Some find the best way to make everyone happ*ier* (no children or husbands are happy all the time), *is to be happy first, just within yourself, just for yon.* After all, frequently the things that seem the most complicated are actually quite simple: if we want things to change, we need to, you know, change. If what we're doing isn't working, rather than repeating the pattern and expecting a different result, we can make an opposite choice and see what occurs. You might just make some magic happen, Mama!

It may take a few days to a week for everyone in the house to respond to your changes. Many moms say if you start forgetting to make those deliberate external choices, things will quickly slide, but the reality is *the mother sets the tone*. Just another example of how much power women *do* have to control their environments, even when things seem like they're in a state of chaos.

Many moms also say appreciating all the good you yourself are doing for the family, as well as the good things your partner is doing, rather than just observing what he (or you) is/are *not* doing at home, can help a woman "not feel like choking her husband. At least not as often," according to one mom of two.

Bottom line? Sometimes it's more peaceful for both of you to ease up on "understanding each other," in the postpartum period. You are allowed to take a page from Grandma's Book of Wisdom, and just smile, give dad the three-sentence summary of the day, confidently, yet kindly, give him a quantifiable task or two (he can learn the "Family Man" thing, it just takes time and patience...), then go call someone with two X chromosomes who gets it. You can catch up with him later over a bowl of ice cream (you could both use some fun together!), and don't worry, you'll like him again. There's just no cure for being a man.

Total Exhaustion

Nearly every new mom expects to be "tired," but few of us have any clue what total, desperate exhaustion feels like (and how we will cope or not cope) until we are eyeball-deep in it and drowning. As a new mom you can expect to be completely exhausted. If you're not, you are fortunate, but don't talk about it too much–you will alienate all the other exhausted moms around you. One mother said this about postpartum exhaustion:

> With my first baby I kept expecting to catch up on sleep and somehow feel rested during those first 6 weeks. I wish I had just accepted that it isn't possible, and that living with exhaustion is just going to be norm for a while. Maybe others could put it better, but this was a huge thing for me.
>
> ELENA B.

One more thing related to exhaustion. This was touched on in Chapter 3: Trying to Sleep at the Hospital, but it bears repeating. If you start having thoughts that worry or scare you, reach out for help immediately. Get a referral from your provider for a mental-health professional *who is experienced in perinatal/postpartum mental health complications.* You are likely experiencing "intrusive thoughts," a common, and often terrifying symptom of Post-partum Obsessive-Compulsive Disorder (OCD).

Postpartum OCD is an expression of Postpartum Distress and is frequently triggered by exhaustion/sleep deprivation. Women who experience this symptom often fear they are "going crazy," but remember this—if you're *afraid* you're going crazy, you're probably not *actually going* crazy. If the scary thoughts seem to make sense to you and you are in the midst of making a *plan* to act on the scary thoughts, that would be different. That would be a sign of *postpartum psychosis, an extremely serious perinatal mental health complication that requires immediate medical attention.*

Please know this: *no matter how bad things ever seem, it is never hopeless.* All postpartum mental-health issues are highly treatable if addressed. Do not conceal your true feelings and worries. If you are having thoughts that scare you, please reach out for help immediately. You can go to www.postpartum. net and find local help from providers who understand. You are not alone, no matter how you feel. There is help. *You are not alone.*

An Identity Crisis

Some women feel a loss of themselves when they become mothers. One new mom said:

It seemed like all the best parts of me were gone. I wasn't considerate, funny, thoughtful, interesting, intelligent, attractive, or even nice. I tried to be those things, but I felt like I was running on ice. I couldn't even think.

I was in so much pain post-birth, but it seemed like I was supposed to be happy, and I didn't want to be a downer, so I just pretended everything was great. It was truly exhausting, and frightening, too. I felt so alone—like I had a terrible secret, and didn't know how long I could keep up the charade of pretending to be my former self.

What's worse, I was sure once everyone in my life found out how inept I was, they'd turn away from me. I felt that after all these great expectations people had of me being a good person, and good mother. I was going to let everybody down.

LAURA W.

Some new moms are shocked to find that they feel a loss of their own identities when they become mothers. Whether it's because a woman is no longer at work and spending time with friends like she used to, or because she is thrust into a new peer group of "mommies"—with whom she may or may not have anything in common aside from having babies—it can be pretty tough to take on this new role of "mom" and try to shove yourself into some foreign idea of what that means. It takes time to find that new sense of self. If you're having a hard time with this, it's not just you, and it does get better.

Feeling a loss of identity can be a sign of Post-partum Distress. Many new moms experiencing identity loss or confusion have found a lot of comfort and encouragement in postpartum/new-mom-peer-support groups. You can reach out and contact www.postpartumflorida.org, www.postpartum.net or other local postpartum-peer-support resources in your area. To quote one mom from one of our support groups, "What a difference venting and some conversation with other understanding women can make!"

Postpartum Stress and Distress

What kicked me this time around was L's intensity first and foremost, and that led me to not having any time to spend with my 2-year-old. I was so incredibly resentful of him because he took me away from my daughter. Finally, I got on board with a great therapist—rather later than I should have—and things got better.

Objectively, life is easier now because the little man is mellowing out slowly, but surely. We also build in one-on-one time for the girl and me, even if Baby L screams his head off the whole time. Having a paid professional for me to talk to has been super helpful, too.

ANGIE G.

Rarely does a woman plan on having Postpartum Distress (Depression, Anxiety, or OCD), but it is the most common complication of childbirth, affecting up to one out of every three new mothers. Moms who experience Postpartum Distress often say they wish they'd known how to identify it in themselves, how common it actually is, and how many resources there are for help.

Over the last eight years as a mother, friend, and Peer Support Group facilitator, I've observed a pattern of "shock-fear-stress-distress" among new moms. The initial shock of an unexpected issue leads to fear. (Because the issue is new, we don't fully understand it, and we are afraid of what we don't understand.) Then, in a state of fear, which is when we make our worst decisions. We react. This reaction leads to stress (because our fear-based reaction was predictably lousy), which leads to distress because we still have a scary new problem we've just made a little worse, and the ship begins to sink. Now the postpartum mom likely feels afraid, out of control, and a deep sense of failure because "a good mother would know what to do," we unreasonably scold ourselves.

The downward spiral of "worry-fear-doubt-failure" begins, and if left uninterrupted, intensifies in an already exhausted mother's mind. Anxiety takes over unchecked, hopelessness sets in, and if unaddressed, the new mother can find herself in a mental and emotional crater known as Postpartum Distress. Postpartum Distress is a broad term for Postpartum Mood and Anxiety Disorders, which includes Postpartum Anxiety, Depression, Obsessive-Compulsive Disorder, Panic, and more. The above progression is just one row of dominos to Postpartum Distress, but a very common one.

If you are feeling any of the following, you are not alone, and you may be experiencing one or more expressions of Postpartum Distress, including Depression and/or Anxiety:

I feel...

- ♥ Scared
- ♥ Angry
- ♥ Out of control

Or like:

- ♥ I'm never going to feel like myself again.
- ♥ Each day is 100 hours long.
- ♥ No one understands.
- ♥ My relationship cannot survive this.
- ♥ I'm a bad mother.
- ♥ I should never have had this baby.
- ♥ Every little thing gets on my nerves.

- ♥ If I could get a good night's sleep, everything would be okay.
- ♥ I have no patience for anything anymore.
- ♥ I'm going crazy.
- ♥ I will always feel like this.

If you are feeling any of the above, you are not alone,, it is not your fault, and with support you will be well.

Right now is the time for you to reach out for support as soon as you can, and talk and keep talking to someone you can trust: your partner, mother, friends, the pediatrician, a childbirth educator you liked, your lactation consultant, or visit www.post-partum.net, the website of Postpartum Support International, one of the most established and reliable postpartum-support organizations in the world, to find local postpartum support and resources in your community.

Again, the key is to *talk to someone you trust*. It is normal to feel exhausted or overwhelmed at times, but it is not okay for you to be suffering with feelings or moods that frighten you, or to be struggling to care of your baby and/or yourself. Postpartum Distress is real and terrifying, but highly treatable, and you do not have to put up with that kind of torture. It is not your fault. You do not deserve to feel that way. You are a good mother to see that something is wrong, and even though the whole motherhood situation may seem hopeless, with the support you need, *you will feel better.**

Note: If you are having thoughts about hurting yourself or your baby, get help immediately. Please see below for resources.

If you, or anyone you know, needs immediate assistance, please use one of the following resources:

EMERGENCY: 911

SUICIDE PREVENTION HOTLINE: 1-800-273-TALK (8255)

The postpartum period is so complicated, far more complicated than many women ever could have imagined. Like snowflakes, no two postpartum experiences are alike, and it only makes sense that each woman needs a specific combination of support as she transitions to motherhood. As one first-time mom said:

> *I thought becoming a mother was going to be all about taking care of "the baby." I had no earthly clue what it was going to do to me! Now 7 years and three children later, I really get it—9 months to get to baby, and at least a year to get a new self. It is the biggest of big deals.*

> LAURA W.

Postpartum Distress is about many, many factors. Being honest and reaching out for help can turn a tough situation around, and often faster than you think. No matter what comes up in your postpartum experience, just remember: *there are people who can help.* Understanding support is always one call (or a few keystrokes) away.

Finding the "New Normal"

> *In all likelihood everything really will be okay, but, as many new moms wish someone had told them, there is no "getting back to normal." You and your partner–and your baby–will find a "new normal."*

As mentioned before, your own physical, mental, and emotional recovery, and as well as your adjustment to being responsible for an innocent, defenseless little person, is going to take time and patience, and a sense of humor, too. In all likelihood, everything will shake out fine. Still, the truth that many new moms wish someone had told them is there really is no "getting back to normal." You, your partner, and your baby will find a crazy, authentic, one-of-a-kind "new normal."

A last word from a mom of four, survivor of Postpartum Depression/Anxiety, and Postpartum Society of Florida SISTER Support volunteer on adjusting to motherhood:

You are exactly the mom your baby needs. Hang in there—early motherhood can be a wild ride, but there are great women out there who get it and can relate to whatever you're going through. Be kind to yourself, you will find your way, and above all remember, dear Mama: you are not alone!

BARBARA T.

Time to Fly

Well, amazing Mama, you've now read the secret scoop on everything that goes down from your birth to baby's first birthday (a.k.a., your graduation from Mommy Bootcamp). I hope you now feel ready to "expect the unexpected" as you enter one of the most beautiful, intense, and indescribable periods of your life. The upside of any experience related to babies is that good, bad, or ugly, it's bound to change, and though it's a steep learning curve, you'll be an outstanding mom. Just the fact that you care enough to read books about preparing for motherhood shows how devoted you are to giving yourself and your baby a good strong start.

As a matter of fact, feel free to repeatedly tell yourself what a good mother you are. Your baby can't say it (and can't even smile at you for the first couple months—tough stuff if you thrive on feedback), and your partner won't always say it even if he's thinking it (side effect of being a man). So moms need to be their own best advocates. Say it to yourself during the long, dark nights, especially from weeks 3 to 12, but beyond, too.

- ❤ I am a good mother.
- ❤ I am working really hard.
- ❤ This will get easier.
- ❤ I am a good mother and we're going to be okay.

And FYI—the second year of life with your child, when sleep is more settled, and you can start having adventures together, is much more fun, and can be such a treasured reward after the intensity of the first.

Birthing and raising a baby is really, really hard work. The hardest work there is for the body, heart, and soul, and also the most special. After my first baby was born, I was blown away by the enormity of the big picture of parenthood. I'd had happy images of life as a mother, but when reality hit, it was really overwhelming to be "the mom!" Yes, parenthood is life-changing, to say the least:time, energy, patience, devotion, attention, understanding. Everything! But the relationships are built just one moment at a time.

Raising a child is the investment that reaps rewards throughout, and far beyond, your lifetime. I wish you and yours only the best. Please get in touch anytime, and most of all—congratulations!!!

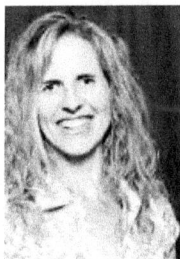

ABOUT THE AUTHOR

Sarah Workman Checcone is the
founder and Executive Director
of Postpartum Society of Florida
(www.postpartumflorida.org),
a non-profit mom-to-mom organi-
zation based in Sarasota, whose mission is to ease the
transition from pregnancy to parenthood. She holds
a Juris Doctor in Law degree from the University of
Miami, and a Bachelor of Fine Arts degree in Musical
Theatre from the University of Michigan.

Sarah is also a Certified Instructor of the Myers-Briggs
Type Indicator® and the MMTIC®. Sarah loves to
sing, laugh, eat delicious food someone else cooked,
be outside, encourage amazing women, and hang out
with her husband and four cutie kiddos.

POSTPARTUM SOCIETY OF FLORIDA

www.ingramcontent.com/pod-product-compliance
Lightning Source LLC
Chambersburg PA
CBHW050559280326
41933CB00011B/1908